Table of Contents

Introduction

Eating is essential to life. Many of us look to eating as not only a necessity, but also a pleasure. You may have been told since childhood to start the day with a good breakfast to give you the energy to get through most of the day. You most likely have heard about the importance of a balanced diet, with plenty of fruits and vegetables. But what does this all mean to your body and the physiological processes it carries out each day? You need to absorb a range of nutrients so that your cells have the building blocks for metabolic processes that release the energy for the cells to carry out their daily jobs, to manufacture new proteins, cells, and body parts, and to recycle materials in the cell. This chapter will take you through some of the chemical reactions essential to life, the sum of which is referred to as metabolism. The focus of these discussions will be anabolic reactions and catabolic reactions. You will examine the various chemical reactions that are important to sustain life, including why you must have oxygen, how mitochondria transfer energy, and the importance of certain "metabolic" hormones and vitamins. Metabolism varies, depending on age, gender, activity level, fuel consumption, and lean body mass. Your own metabolic rate fluctuates throughout life. By modifying your diet and exercise regimen, you can increase both lean body mass and metabolic rate. Factors affecting metabolism also play important roles in controlling muscle mass. Aging is known to decrease the metabolic rate by as much as 5 percent per year. Additionally, because men tend have more lean muscle mass then women, their basal metabolic rate (metabolic rate at rest) is higher; therefore, men tend to burn more calories than women do. Lastly, an individual's inherent metabolic rate is a function of the proteins and enzymes derived from their genetic background. Thus, your genes play a big role in your metabolism. Nonetheless, each person's body engages in the same overall metabolic processes. Metabolic processes are constantly taking place in the body. Metabolism is the sum of all of the chemical reactions that are involved in catabolism and anabolism. The reactions governing the breakdown of food to obtain energy are called catabolic reactions. Conversely, anabolic reactions use the energy produced by catabolic reactions to synthesize larger molecules from smaller ones, such as when the body forms proteins by stringing together amino acids. Both sets of reactions are critical to maintaining life. Because catabolic reactions produce energy and anabolic reactions use energy, ideally, energy usage would balance the energy produced. If the net energy change is positive (catabolic reactions release more energy than the anabolic reactions use), then the body stores the excess energy by building fat molecules for long-term storage. On the other hand, if the net energy change is negative (catabolic reactions release less energy than anabolic reactions use), the body uses stored energy to compensate for the deficiency of energy released by catabolism.

What is Metabolism?

Metabolism is a term that is used to describe all chemical reactions involved in maintaining the living state of the cells and the organism. Metabolism can be conveniently divided into two categories:

Catabolism - the breakdown of molecules to obtain energy

Anabolism - the synthesis of all compounds needed by the cells

Metabolism is closely linked to nutrition and the availability of nutrients. Bioenergetics is a term that describes the biochemical or metabolic pathways by which the cell ultimately obtains energy. Energy formation is one of the vital components of metabolism.

Nutrition, Metabolism and Energy

Nutrition is the key to metabolism. The pathways of metabolism rely upon nutrients that they breakdown in order to produce energy. This energy in turn is required by the body to synthesize molecules like new proteins and nucleic acids (DNA, RNA).

Nutrients in relation to metabolism encompass factors like bodily requirements for various substances, individual functions in the body, the amount needed, and the level below which poor health results.

Essential nutrients supply energy (calories) and supply the necessary chemicals which the body itself cannot synthesize. Food provides a variety of substances that are essential for the building, upkeep, and repair of body tissues, and for the efficient functioning of the body.

The diet needs essential nutrients like carbon, hydrogen, oxygen, nitrogen, phosphorus, sulfur, and around 20 other inorganic elements. The major elements are supplied in carbohydrates, lipids, and protein. In addition, vitamins, minerals and water are necessary.

Carbohydrates in Metabolism

Foods supply carbohydrates in three forms: starch, sugar, and cellulose (fiber). Starches and sugars form major and essential sources of energy for humans. Fibers contribute to bulk in diet.

Body tissues depend on glucose for all activities. Carbohydrates and sugars yield glucose by digestion or metabolism.

The overall reaction for the combustion of glucose is written as:

$C_6H_{12}O_6 + 6\ O_2 \longrightarrow 6\ CO_2 + 6\ H_2O + energy$

Most people consume around half of their diet as carbohydrates. This comes from foods such as rice, wheat, bread, potatoes and pasta.

Proteins in Metabolism

Proteins are the main tissue builders in the body. They are part of every cell in the body. Proteins help in cell structure, functions, hemoglobin formation to carry oxygen, enzymes to carry out vital reactions and a myriad of other functions in the body. Proteins are also vital in supplying nitrogen for DNA and RNA genetic material and energy production. Proteins are necessary for nutrition because they contain amino acids. Among the 20 or more amino acids, the human body is unable to synthesize 8 and these are called essential amino acids.

The essential amino acids include:

Lysine

Tryptophan

Methionine

Leucine

Isoleucine

Phenylalanine

Valine

Threonine

Foods with the best quality protein are eggs, milk, soybeans, meats, vegetables, and grains.

Fat in Metabolism

Fats are concentrated sources of energy. They produce twice as much energy as either carbohydrates or protein on a weight basis.

The functions of fats include:

Helping to form the cellular structure;

Forming a protective cushion and insulation around vital organs;

Helping absorb fat-soluble vitamins,

Providing a reserve storage for energy

Essential fatty acids include unsaturated fatty acids like linoleic, linolenic, and arachidonic acids. These need to be taken in diet. Saturated fats, along with cholesterol, have been implicated in arteriosclerosis and heart disease.

Minerals and Vitamins in Metabolism

The minerals in foods do not contribute directly to energy needs but are important as body regulators and play a role in metabolic pathways of the body. More than 50 elements are found in the human body. About 25 elements have been found to be essential, meaning a deficiency produces specific deficiency symptoms.

Important minerals include:

Calcium

Phosphorus

Iron

Sodium

Potassium

Chloride ions

Copper

Cobalt

Manganese

Zinc

Magnesium

Fluorine

Iodine

Vitamins are essential organic compounds that the human body cannot synthesize by itself and must, therefore, be present in the diet. Vitamins particularly important in metabolism include:

Vitamin A

B2 (riboflavin)

Niacin or nicotinic acid

Pantothenic Acid

Metabolic Pathways

The chemical reactions of metabolism are organized into metabolic pathways. These allow the basic chemicals from nutrition to be transformed through a series of steps into another chemical, by a sequence of enzymes.

Enzymes are crucial to metabolism because they allow organisms to drive desirable reactions that require energy. These reactions also are coupled with those that release energy. As enzymes act as catalysts they allow these reactions to proceed quickly and efficiently. Enzymes also allow the regulation of metabolic pathways in response to changes in the cell's environment or signals from other cells.

How a Metabolic Diet Works: Increasing Your Metabolism

If you have a baseline metabolic rate giving you a certain amount of calories needed per day, plus some extra to help you do your daily activities, then what if you could speed up that rate and use your caloric intake more efficiently? We could then burn through all those stored calories in our fat deposits.

Doctors, scientists, and many others have studied this for years, hoping to find a way to help increase an individual's metabolic rate through different foods, supplements, exercise. From this, several diets have emerged over the decades. Their premise is that if you follow their rules or guidelines, you can increase your metabolism and convert the food you eat into energy instead of storing it as fat.

The Metabolic Typing Diet

Metabolism is classified in 3 ways: fast oxidizer, slow oxidizer, and mixed oxidizer (Dominant Protein type, Dominant Carb type, and mixed protein-carb type). It is determined by your autonomic nervous system and your rate of oxidation. The book gives readers a test to assess their Metabolic Type and then follow the plan that fits them the best. This is a major red flag as this diet is supposed to be based on the autonomic nervous system and a BMR rate test that are not valuations you can make through a test written in a book.

The actual plan includes five smaller meals throughout the day that are no more than 4 hours apart, supposedly to avoid blood sugar spikes and cravings. All refined and processed carbohydrates should be eliminated. Dairy, soy, alcohol, and caffeine intake should be limited as well.

There are differing studies that show benefits for or harm to weight loss goals by frequent meals. The idea of small regular meals can go against the new research coming out about the benefits of intermittent fasting for weight loss and burning fat. Studies showed no difference in weight loss by the number of meals eaten per day.

Indeed, with more frequent eating, it stands to reason that the body has to release more insulin throughout the day to handle the incoming meals. Therefore, it cannot fully recover back to baseline until the end of the day, which is generally the most significant meal. Some reviews state that the evidence is inconclusive for the optimal meal frequency for weight loss and that a reduced meal frequency can lead to improved lipid panels. The Metabolic Typing Diet has a host of issues starting from a vague categorization of Metabolic Type leading to a prescribed way of eating that has no scientific basis for weight loss.

40% carbohydrates + 30% protein + 30% fat

The benefit of the Zone Diet is that you can follow this formula in any setting, at any restaurant, or any takeaway meal. You can cook this way and batch prepare foods that fit into the buckets, and essentially, you can follow this for the rest of your life. The categories are broad enough that you won't feel bored or boxed in by the same chicken + brown rice + broccoli meal day in and day out.

Lean proteins can be anything from turkey, chicken, pork, fish, shellfish, tofu, and egg whites. Low glycemic carbs can be fruits like berries, apples, oranges; veggies like asparagus, broccoli, cucumber, tomatoes, zucchini; and beans, chickpeas, lentils, wild rice. Examples of monounsaturated fats are found in oils like olive oil, as well as avocados and most nuts.

The other benefit of the Zone Diet is that there is no caloric limit, only the macro allocation per meal. Some people find this more flexible and liberating than constantly tracking points or calories like other popular diets.

The Atkins Diet

The Atkins Diet is a trendy diet created and it was vilified for a while due to its reliance on a large amount of fat in the diet, but subsequent research has shown that not all fat is bad, and in fact, it can be pretty essential to a healthy diet.

There are 4 phases to the Atkins Diet, and the first phase is very similar to a ketogenic diet:

Phase 1 or Induction

20 grams of carbs per day for two weeks. Focus on fat and protein, with some low glycemic veggies on the side. This phase is designed to promote weight loss.

Phase 2 or Balancing

Gradually adding in nuts and other lower glycemic carbs like veggies and fruits.

Phase 3 or Fine-tuning

Approach your goal weight and continue to add carbs to your diet until weight loss slows down.

Phase 4 or Maintenance = this is the "lifestyle" part of the diet where you can eat as many low glycemic carbs as your body can handle without increasing weight.

Again, similar to the Zone Diet, this diet does not rely on counting calories and promotes the kinds of foods that many people find to be satiating because they are high in fat and protein.

Are these Diets Safe for Everyone?

These diets are meant to be guidelines for a lifestyle and are designed to help people change their nutrition choices for the better and the rest of their lives. These are dietary guidelines that work well for those willing to invest and put the work in to follow these rules over a significant time.

As mentioned above, these diets or dietary patterns promote foods higher in protein and fats, which are naturally satiating. Therefore, people tend to feel full with smaller portions or feel full overall, something they may have lost while following a higher carbohydrate diet. That feeling of fullness can help curb sweets cravings and snacking between meals, leading to excess caloric intake and weight gain.

However, while there are no significant inherent risks with these diets on a short-term basis (<6 months), there may be risks associated with following any of these restrictive diets on a long-term basis. The more restrictive a diet is, the greater the possibility for nutrient deficiencies. This does not mean restrictive diets cannot be done properly and healthily, but more attention to detail is required for long-term success. Finally, for some people long-term restriction can lead to increased feelings of cravings and subsequent binge eating.

Therefore, the people who will have the most success following one of these diets, are those who are willing to make sure that they are supplementing where needed and keeping an eye on those micro or macronutrients where they might be under or overdoing it.

Always consult your doctor before starting a metabolic-related diet or any other diet, especially if you have pre-existing conditions like diabetes.

Metabolic flexibility is critical in keeping your glucose at healthy levels.

Without monitoring your glucose levels, you can never truly see the response your body has to any dietary or lifestyle changes you make.

If you want to take a big step towards metabolic health, the NutriSense Continuous Glucose Health Program can provide you with a combination of leading CGM technology and personalized support from Registered Dietitians. The program makes monitoring and understanding glucose simple so that you can take charge of your metabolic health.

Try it for yourself to analyze your glucose levels and meet your health goals.

The 12 Best Foods to Boost Your Metabolism

If you're trying to lose weight or maintain your weight, you might be looking for foods that can boost your metabolism.

It's true that certain foods may help slightly increase your metabolic rate. This is the number of calories that your body burns.

Adding these foods to your diet may make it slightly easier to lose body fat or prevent excess weight gain, if that's your goal.

However, eating more of these foods doesn't guarantee you'll lose weight. Instead, they serve as a complement to a balanced, moderately calorie-restricted diet to promote weight loss.

Here are 12 foods that may rev up your metabolism.

1. Protein-rich foods

Protein-rich foods — such as meat, fish, eggs, dairy, legumes, nuts, and seeds — could help increase your metabolism for a few hours.

This is because they require your body to use more energy to digest them. This is known as the thermic effect of food (TEF).

The TEF refers to the number of calories your body needs to digest, absorb, and process the nutrients in your meals.

Research shows that protein-rich foods increase TEF the most. For example, they increase your metabolic rate by 15–30%, compared with 5–10% for carbs and 0–3% for fats (1).

Protein-rich diets also reduce the drop in metabolism often seen during weight loss by helping your body hold on to its muscle mass.

What's more, protein may also help keep you fuller for longer, which can prevent overeating.

2. Mineral-Rich Foods

The minerals iron and selenium each play different but equally important roles in the proper functioning of your body.

However, they do have one thing in common. They're both required for the proper functioning of your thyroid gland, which regulates your metabolism.

Research shows that a diet too low in iron or selenium may reduce your thyroid's ability to produce sufficient amounts of hormones, which could slow down your metabolism.

To help your thyroid function to the best of its ability, include selenium- and iron-rich foods like meat, seafood, legumes, nuts, and seeds in your daily menu.

3. Chili Peppers

Capsaicin, a chemical found in chili peppers, may boost your metabolism by slightly increasing the rate at which your body burns calories.

In fact, a review of 20 research studies notes that capsaicin — from supplements or the peppers themselves — may help your body burn around 50 extra calories per day.

Some studies report similar benefits with doses as low as 9–10 mg per day. This is equivalent to one jalapeño pepper.

Moreover, capsaicin may have appetite-reducing properties.

According to a review of studies in nearly 200 people, consuming at least 2 mg of capsaicin directly before each meal appears to reduce calorie consumption, especially from carbs.

Similarly, adding cayenne pepper to your meal may increase the amount of fat your body burns for energy, especially following a high fat meal. However, this fat-burning effect may only apply to people unaccustomed to consuming spicy foods.

That said, findings are mixed on capsaicin's metabolism-boosting abilities.

4. Coffee

The caffeine found in coffee may help increase metabolic rate.

Several studies have noted that people who consume at least 270 mg of caffeine daily, or the equivalent of about 3 cups of coffee, burn up to an extra 100 calories per day.

Furthermore, caffeine may help your body burn fat for energy, and it seems especially effective at boosting your workout performance.

However, its effects vary from person to person, based on individual characteristics such as body weight and age.

5. Tea

Tea contains health-boosting compounds called catechins that may work in tandem with caffeine to boost metabolic rate.

In particular, both oolong and matcha green tea may increase fat oxidation and may help you burn extra calories when part of an exercise plan.

In addition, oolong and green teas may help your body use stored fat for energy more effectively, increasing your fat-burning ability by up to 17%.

Nevertheless, as is the case with coffee, effects may vary from person to person.

6. Beans and Legumes

Legumes and beans — such as lentils, peas, chickpeas, black beans, and peanuts — are particularly high in protein compared to other plant foods.

Studies suggest that their high protein content requires your body to burn more calories to digest them, compared to lower-protein foods. This is due to their TEF.

Legumes also contain dietary fiber, including resistant starch and soluble fiber, which your body can use as a prebiotic to feed the good bacteria living in your large intestine.

In turn, these friendly bacteria produce short-chain fatty acids, which may help your body more effectively use stored fat as energy and maintain normal blood sugar levels.

7. Ginger

Ginger and related spices are thought to have particularly beneficial metabolism-boosting properties.

For instance, research shows that dissolving 2 grams of ginger powder in hot water and drinking it with a meal may help you burn up to 43 more calories than drinking hot water alone.

This hot ginger drink also may decrease levels of hunger and enhance feelings of satiety (fullness).

Grains of paradise, another spice in the ginger family, may have similar effects.

A study in 19 healthy males reported that participants given a 40 mg extract of grains of paradise burned 43 more calories in the following 2 hours than those given a placebo.

That said, researchers also noted that some of the participants were non-responders, so the effects may vary from one person to another.

8. Cacao

Cacao and cocoa are tasty treats that may also benefit your metabolism.

For instance, studies in mice have noted that cocoa and cocoa extracts may promote the expression of genes that stimulate fat burning. This appears to especially true in mice fed high fat or high calorie diets.

Interestingly, one study suggests that cocoa may prevent the action of enzymes necessary to break down fat and carbs during digestion, which could prevent the body from absorbing them and the calories they provide.

However, human studies examining the effects of cocoa, cacao, or cacao products like dark chocolate are rare. More studies are needed before strong conclusions can be drawn.

If you'd like to give cacao a try, opt for raw versions. Processing tends to reduce the amounts of beneficial compounds and add extra sugar and calories.

9. Apple cider vinegar

Apple cider vinegar may increase your metabolism.

Animal studies have shown vinegar to be particularly helpful in increasing the amount of fat burned for energy. Likewise, apple cider vinegar is often claimed to boost metabolism in humans, but few studies have investigated this directly. It may help you lose weight by slowing stomach emptying and enhancing feelings of fullness.

If you decide to take it, make sure to limit yourself to 1–2 tablespoons per day and dilute it in at least 1 cup of water per tablespoon of vinegar to limit the risk of tooth erosion, damage to the lining of your digestive tract, or other potential side effects.

10. Medium chain triglyceride (MCT) oil

MCT oil is a unique type of fat that may offer some metabolic benefits. Most fats found in foods are long-chain triglycerides, but MCT oil is comprised of medium-chain triglycerides.

Some studies have shown that MCT oil consumption can increase metabolic rate in humans. Additionally, unlike long-chain fats, once MCTs are absorbed, they go directly to the liver to be turned into energy. This makes them less likely to be stored as body fat.

MCT oil is typically taken as a supplement, although it can be added to foods like soups or smoothies. It's not suitable for cooking, though.

11. Water

Drinking enough water is a great way to stay hydrated. Additionally, some studies show that drinking water may also briefly boost metabolism by 24–30%.

Researchers note that about 40% of that increase is explained by the additional calories needed to heat the water to body temperature — known as water induced thermogenesis.

However, the effects only appear to last for 40–90 minutes after drinking water, and the strength of the effect may vary from person to person.

12. Seaweed

Seaweed is rich in iodine, a mineral required for the production of thyroid hormones and proper functioning of your thyroid gland.

Thyroid hormones have various functions, one of which is to regulate your metabolic rate.

Regularly consuming seaweed can help you meet your iodine needs and maintain your metabolic health.

What's more, fucoxanthin is another seaweed-based compound — primarily found in brown seaweeds — that may increase your metabolic rate.

Metabolism Diet Recipes

Savory Diet Chicken

Very simple, healthy and delicious! The amounts are up to you! (Note: As a general guide, one serving would consist of one chicken breast with 1 to 2 of each of the vegetables). Easy and flexible!

Ingredients

4 skinless, boneless chicken breast halves

6 potatoes

2 green bell peppers, sliced

1 cup cubed carrots

2 onions, quartered

1 dash Worcestershire sauce

1 teaspoon paprika

Directions

Step 1

Preheat oven to 350 degrees F (175 degrees C).

Step 2

In a 9x13 inch baking dish, place the chicken breasts. Add the potatoes, bell peppers, carrot and onion, all cubed or quartered. Sprinkle all liberally with Worcestershire sauce and a dash of paprika. Cover dish and bake in the preheated oven for 1 1/2 hour. That's it! Enjoy!

Nutrition Facts

Per Serving: 425 calories; protein 35.2g; carbohydrates 67.1g; fat 2.1g; cholesterol 68.4mg; sodium 123mg.

Keto Diet Avocado Egg Bake

Keto designed egg and avocado breakfast for 1.

Ingredients

1 avocado, halved and pitted

2 eggs

¼ cup shredded Cheddar cheese

salt and freshly ground black pepper to taste

1 tablespoon chopped fresh parsley, or to taste (Optional)

Directions

Step 1

Preheat the oven to 425 degrees F (220 degrees C).

Step 2

Scoop out a little of the avocado from where the pit was to make room for 1 egg. Place on a baking sheet and crack 1 egg on top of each avocado half.

Step 3

Bake in the preheated oven until egg is cooked, 15 to 20 minutes. Sprinkle Cheddar cheese on top and season with salt and pepper. Garnish with fresh parsley.

Nutrition Facts

Per Serving: 605 calories; protein 25.3g; carbohydrates 18.6g; fat 50.9g; cholesterol 408.2mg; sodium 525.4mg.

DASH Diet Mexican Bake

Mexican flavors will make this chicken casserole a family favorite.

Ingredients

1½ cups cooked rice, preferably brown

1 pound skinless, boneless chicken breast, cut in bite-sized pieces

2 (14.5 ounce) cans no-salt-added tomatoes, diced or crushed

1 (15 ounce) can no-salt-added black beans, drained and rinsed

1 cup frozen yellow corn kernels

1 cup chopped red bell pepper

1 cup chopped poblano pepper

1 tablespoon chili powder

1 tablespoon cumin

4 garlic cloves, crushed

1 cup shredded reduced-fat Monterey Jack cheese

¼ cup jalapeno pepper slices (Optional)

Directions

Step 1

Preheat oven to 400 degrees. Spread rice in a shallow 3-quart casserole. Top with chicken. In a bowl, combine tomatoes, beans, corn, peppers, seasonings and garlic; pour over chicken. Top with cheese and optional jalapeno. Bake 45 minutes.

Nutrition Facts

Per Serving: 325 calories; protein 28.4g; carbohydrates 36.9g; fat 7.1g; cholesterol 56.5mg; sodium 355.8mg.

Keto Diet Low Carb Pancakes

Delicious, easy, and quick keto pancakes. Serve with syrup and customize with your choice of toppings, like pecans, whipped cream, or blueberry jam. If you are strictly Keto, leave out the sugar.

Ingredients

2 ounces cream cheese, softened

2 eggs

1 teaspoon white sugar

½ teaspoon ground cinnamon

Cooking spray

Directions

Step 1

Combine cream cheese, eggs, sugar, and cinnamon in a blender; blend until smooth. Let rest 2 minutes or lightly tap on counter to remove bubbles.

Step 2

Heat a skillet over medium heat and grease with cooking spray. Pour 1/4 of the batter into the skillet; cook until bubbles start to form, about 2 minutes. Flip and cook until cooked through, about 1 minute. Transfer to a clean plate. Repeat with remaining batter.

Nutrition Facts

Per Serving: 362 calories; protein 16.9g; carbohydrates 7.4g; fat 30g; cholesterol 434.4mg; sodium 307.9mg.

Chocolate Chip Cookies for Special Diets

Be sure to use a heat-stable sugar substitute. Since the substitutes vary in strength, use an amount equal to 3/4 cup regular sugar according to the package.

Ingredients

½ cup butter, softened

¾ cup granulated artificial sweetener

2 tablespoons water

½ teaspoon vanilla extract

1 egg beaten

1cup all-purpose flour

½ teaspoon baking soda

½ teaspoon salt

½ cup semisweet chocolate chips

½ cup chopped pecans

Directions

Step 1

Preheat oven to 375 degrees F (190 degrees C).

Step 2

In a medium bowl, cream together the butter and sugar substitute. Mix in water, vanilla, and egg. Sift together the flour, baking soda, and salt; stir into the creamed mixture. Mix in the chocolate chips and pecans. Drop cookies by heaping teaspoonfuls onto a cookie sheet.

Step 3

Bake in the preheated oven for 10 to 12 minutes. Remove from cookic shccts to cool on wire racks. These cookies freeze well.

Nutrition Facts

Per Serving: 60 calories; protein 4.2g; carbohydrates 3.5g; fat 3.4g; cholesterol 9mg; sodium 53.8mg.

Spicy Cocoa Almonds

This protein-packed snack is great for healthy eating on the go. The cayenne pepper gives these cocoa almonds a metabolism-boosting kick. Store in an airtight container.

Ingredients

4 cups raw unsalted almonds

2 tablespoons unsweetened cocoa powder

1 teaspoon granular sucralose sweetener (such as Splenda)

1 teaspoon cayenne pepper (Optional)

Directions

Step 1

Preheat the oven to 350 degrees F (175 degrees C). Place the almonds in a single layer on a rimmed baking tray.

Step 2

Bake in the preheated oven for 5 minutes. Stir and continue baking until fragrant and toasty, about 5 minutes more. Let cool on tray for 2 minutes; pour into a bowl.

Step 3

Add cocoa powder, sucralose, and cayenne pepper. Stir with a spatula until well coated. Pour almonds back onto the baking tray to cool completely.

Cook's Note:

I like it spicy, but you can use less cayenne or omit altogether if you do not want the heat.

Nutrition Facts

Per Serving: 207 calories; protein 7.7g; carbohydrates 7.4g; fat 18.1g; sodium 0.5mg.

Juicy Slow Cooker Chicken Breast for Any Diet

Super easy, low-fat, and low-calorie chicken breast. Great to set and forget on a busy day. You really can add just about anything to this recipe. I've tried everything from salsa to wine.

Ingredients

1 pound skinless, boneless chicken breast halves

1 (14.5 ounce) can petite diced tomatoes

¼ onion, chopped (Optional)

1 teaspoon Italian seasoning (Optional)

1 clove garlic, minced (Optional)

Directions

Step 1

Arrange chicken in a slow cooker. Pour tomatoes over chicken; add onion, Italian seasoning, and garlic.

Step 2

Cook on Low for 6 to 8 hours.

Cook's Note:

You can use any type of herb in place of the Italian seasoning.

Nutrition Facts

Per Serving: 144 calories; protein 23.1g; carbohydrates 5.2g; fat 2.4g; cholesterol 58.5mg; sodium 208mg.

Bulletproof Hot Chocolate

This is an alternative to Bulletproof® coffee for people following the Bulletproof diet, ketogenic diet, or any high-fat low-carb diet.

Ingredients

11 fluid ounces hot water

2 tablespoons unsalted butter

1 tablespoon medium-chain triglyceride (MCT) oil

1 tablespoon cacao powder

1 tablespoon cacao butter

? teaspoon vanilla powder

6 drops liquid stevia, or to taste

1 pinch salt

Directions

Step 1

Combine hot water, butter, MCT oil, cacao powder, cacao butter, vanilla powder, liquid stevia, and salt in a blender; blend until smooth.

Cook's Notes:

You can add 1 tablespoon hydrolyzed collagen protein powder and vitamin/supplement powders to the hot chocolate if desired.

I use grass-fed butter. Ghee can also be used in place of the butter, if desired.

Nutrition Facts

Per Serving: 478 calories; protein 3.1g; carbohydrates 9g; fat 50g; cholesterol 61.1mg; sodium 172.1mg.

Keto Vanilla-Cinnamon Cookies

Great cookie for a ketogenic diet.

Ingredients

1 cup almond flour

½ cup finely ground pecans

1 teaspoon cinnamon

½ teaspoon salt

¼ teaspoon ground nutmeg

½ cup butter

¼ cup erythritol

1 egg

1 teaspoon vanilla extract

½ cup coconut flour

Directions

Step 1

Combine almond flour and ground pecans in a skillet over medium heat and cook until golden and fragrant, 3 to 6 minutes. Remove from heat. Whisk cinnamon, salt, and nutmeg into the skillet. Set aside to cool.

Step 2

Combine butter and erythritol in a large bowl; beat using an electric mixer until smooth and creamy. Stir in egg and vanilla extract. Mix in almond flour mixture and coconut flour; stir until dough forms. Form into a roll, wrap in plastic wrap, and refrigerate for 1 hour.

Step 3

Preheat the oven to 350 degrees F (175 degrees C). Line a baking sheet with parchment paper.

Step 4

Cut dough roll into 24 cookies and place on the prepared baking sheet.

Step 5

Bake in the preheated oven until lightly browned, 12 to 15 minutes

Nutrition Facts

Per Serving: 92 calories; protein 1.9g; carbohydrates 5.4g; fat 8.2g; cholesterol 17.9mg; sodium 78.6mg.

Middle Eastern Tomato Salad

This salad is a perfect side dish for any phase of the South Beach Diet, or any other diet for that matter, and it's an incredible tasting summer treat for anyone, whether or not you're on a diet. I think it pairs wonderfully with any kind of grilled meat or fish.

Ingredients

1 cup seeded, finely diced cucumber

1 teaspoon salt

1 cup finely diced tomato

1 cup finely diced sweet onion (such as Vidalia®)

1 cup finely chopped fresh parsley

¾ cup finely chopped mint, or to taste

2 tablespoons olive oil, or more to taste

1 tablespoon fresh lemon juice, or more to taste

salt and ground black pepper to taste

Directions

Step 1

Place diced cucumber into a colander and sprinkle with 1 teaspoon salt or as needed; allow to drain for about 15 minutes. Toss drained cucumber with tomato, sweet onion, parsley, and mint. Drizzle salad with olive oil and fresh lemon juice and season with salt and black pepper. Serve immediately.

Nutrition Facts

Per Serving: 48 calories; protein 0.8g; carbohydrates 4.1g; fat 3.5g; sodium 297.3mg.

Low-Carb Beef Cabbage Stew

I modified another recipe on this site for South Beach Diet Phase 1. Not only is it on my diet, but it tastes delicious! Garnish each serving with sour cream.

Ingredients

2 pounds beef stew meat, trimmed and cut into 1-inch cubes

1 cube beef bouillon

1 cup hot chicken broth

2 large onions, coarsely chopped

1 teaspoon Greek seasoning

¼ teaspoon ground black pepper

2 bay leaves

1 (8 ounce) package shredded cabbage

5 stalks celery, sliced

1 (8 ounce) can whole plum tomatoes, coarsely chopped

1 (8 ounce) can tomato sauce

salt to taste

Directions

Step 1

Cook and stir beef in a large saucepan or Dutch oven until browned, about 5 minutes; drain excess grease.

Step 2

Stir beef bouillon into chicken broth in a bowl until dissolved; add to beef.

Step 3

Mix onions, Greek seasoning, black pepper, and bay leaves into broth-beef mixture; cover saucepan and simmer until beef is tender, about 1 hour 15 minutes. Add cabbage and celery to broth-beef mixture; cover saucepan and simmer until celery is tender, about 30 minutes more.

Step 4

Stir plum tomatoes, tomato sauce, and salt into broth-beef mixture and simmer, uncovered, until stew is slightly thickened, 15 to 20 minutes. Remove and discard bay leaves before serving.

Cook's Note:

Beef broth can be substituted for the chicken broth.

Nutrition Facts

Per Serving: 372 calories; protein 31.8g; carbohydrates 9g; fat 22.7g; cholesterol 99.5mg; sodium 612.1mg.

Eggless Pasta

Anyone on an eggless or low-cholesterol diet will appreciate this recipe.

Ingredients

2 cups semolina flour

½ teaspoon salt

½ cup warm water

Directions

Step 1

In a large bowl, mix flour and salt. Add warm water and stir to make a stiff dough. Increase water if dough seems too dry.

Step 2

Pat the dough into a ball and turn out onto a lightly floured surface. Knead for 10 to 15 minutes. Cover. Let dough rest for 20 minutes.

Step 3

Roll out dough using rolling pin or pasta machine. Work with a 1/4 of the dough at one time. Keep the rest covered, to prevent from drying out. Roll by hand to 1/16 of an inch thick. By machine, stop at the third to last setting.

Step 4

Cut pasta into desired shapes.

Step 5

Cook fresh noodles in boiling salted water for 3 to 5 minutes. Drain.

Nutrition Facts

Per Serving: 301 calories; protein 10.6g; carbohydrates 60.8g; fat 0.9g; sodium 292.4mg.

Chocolate-y Iced Mocha

My favorite morning drink that isn't a diet disaster.

Ingredients

1¼ cups cold coffee, divided

1 envelope low-calorie hot cocoa mix

ice cubes, or as needed

½ cup unsweetened almond milk

2 tablespoons sugar-free chocolate syrup, or more to taste

Directions

Step 1

Heat 1/4 cup coffee in microwave in a mug until warmed, about 30 seconds. Stir cocoa mix into the coffee until dissolved.

Step 2

Fill a large glass with ice cubes. Pour 1 cup cold coffee and almond milk over the ice cubes; stir the cocoa mixture and chocolate syrup into the coffee and almond milk.

Nutrition Facts

Per Serving: 105 calories; protein 5.2g; carbohydrates 16.7g; fat 1.8g; cholesterol 2.9mg; sodium 255.3mg.

Instant Pot Vegan Potato Soup

Just because you choose a vegan diet, doesn't mean food has to be bland. This soup cooks in an Instant Pot, and is tasty even for those who have a normal diet.

Ingredients

1 tablespoon olive oil

1 cup chopped shallots

5 cloves garlic, minced

1½ cups vegetable broth

3½ cups chopped potatoes

1¾ cups cashew milk

2 tablespoons flour

½ teaspoon salt

¼ teaspoon freshly ground black pepper

1/3 cup vegan French onion dip (such as Kite Hill)

2 ounces vegan soy cheddar cheese

2 tablespoons minced fresh chives

Directions

Step 1

Turn on a multi-functional pressure cooker (such as Instant Pot) and select Saute function. Add oil and heat until hot. Add shallots and garlic and saute for 1 minute. Pour in vegetable broth and add potatoes. Cancel Saute mode. Close and lock the lid.

Step 2

Select high pressure according to manufacturer's instructions; set timer for 8 minutes. Allow 10 to 15 minutes for pressure to build.

Step 3

Release pressure using the natural-release method according to manufacturer's instructions, about 8 minutes. Unlock and remove the lid.

Step 4

Meanwhile, stir together cashew beverage and flour in a small microwave-safe bowl until no lumps remain. Microwave for 1 minute, stirring after 30 seconds. Stir into potato mixture. Use a potato masher to mash potatoes down to your preferred thickness. Season with salt and pepper.

Step 5

Mix in vegan French onion dip and stir until well combined. Ladle soup into 4 bowls and top with vegan Cheddar cheese and chives.

Nutrition Facts

Per Serving: 341 calories; protein 7.2g; carbohydrates 35.8g; fat 18.8g; sodium 920.2mg.

Quinoa Dijon and Swiss Burger

Great dish for gluten free and vegetarian diet. Loaded with protein.

Ingredients

1½ cups cooked quinoa

2 tablespoons Dijon mustard

1 egg, beaten

1 clove garlic, minced

2 grinds fresh black pepper

½ cup chickpea (garbanzo bean) flour, or as needed

2 teaspoons vegetable oil, or as needed

2 slices Swiss cheese

Directions

Step 1

Mix quinoa, mustard, egg, garlic, and black pepper together in a bowl; add enough chickpea flour to hold mixture together to form 2 patties.

Step 2

Heat oil in a skillet over medium heat; cook patties in the hot oil until browned and cooked through, about 4 minutes per side. Add a Swiss cheese slice to each patty and warm until cheese melts, 2 to 3 minutes.

Nutrition Facts

Per Serving: 455 calories; protein 21.7g; carbohydrates 48.8g; fat 19.1g; cholesterol 119.1mg; sodium 474.8mg.

Low-Carb Taco Soup

If you are trying Atkins or another low-carb diet...this soup is awesome! This is a perfect recipe for a gluten-free diet as well. Easy to make and delicious. Garnish with cilantro and shredded Cheddar cheese.

Ingredients

3 cups chicken broth, divided

1 small head cauliflower, finely chopped

1 tablespoon olive oil, or as needed

1 onion, finely chopped

1 (4 ounce) can diced jalapeno peppers

1 pound ground beef

1 (8 ounce) package cream cheese, cubed

1 (26 ounce) container diced tomatoes

1 teaspoon ground paprika

Salt and ground black pepper to taste

Directions

Step 1

Combine 2 cups broth and cauliflower in a pot over medium-high heat. Bring to a boil. Reduce heat to medium-low; cook until tender, about 20 minutes.

Step 2

Heat oil in a skillet over medium-high heat. Saute onion and jalapenos until onions are translucent, about 5 minutes. Add beef; cook and stir until browned and crumbly, about 6 minutes.

Step 3

Transfer the cooked cauliflower to a blender and puree. Return to the pot; add cream cheese and remaining 1 cup broth. Cook and stir over medium heat until cream cheese is melted, about 3 minutes. Add the beef mixture, tomatoes, and paprika. Season with salt and pepper. Cook and stir until flavors blend, about 5 minutes.

Nutrition Facts

Per Serving: 377 calories; protein 18.4g; carbohydrates 12.6g; fat 27.6g; cholesterol 90.5mg; sodium 1281.5mg.

Cabbage, Leek, and Broccoli Soup

Just a nice, warming soup - great for diets! Garnish with parsley.

Ingredients

1 tablespoon olive oil

1 onion, thinly sliced

1 leek, thinly sliced

1 potato, cubed

½ cup broccoli florets

Cup shredded cabbage

2 cups vegetable broth

Salt and freshly ground black pepper to taste

Directions

Step 1

Heat oil in a saucepan over medium heat. Add onion and leek; cook and stir until translucent, about 5 minutes. Stir in potato, broccoli, and cabbage. Reduce heat to medium-low and cook, stirring occasionally, until softened, 3 to 5 minutes.

Step 2

Pour vegetable broth into the saucepan. Bring to a boil; reduce heat and simmer until vegetables are tender, about 15 minutes. Season with salt and pepper.

Nutrition Facts

Per Serving: 255 calories; protein 5.9g; carbohydrates 42.7g; fat 7.7g; sodium 567.2mg.

Baked Spinach and Egg White Muffins

These 'muffins' can be eaten warm or cold and are an Atkins Diet-friendly option.

Ingredients

Cooking spray

2 tablespoons olive oil

2 cups fresh spinach, or to taste

12 egg whites

2 egg yolks

1 tablespoon grated Parmesan cheese

1 tablespoon shredded Mexican cheese blend

1 teaspoon garlic powder

¼ teaspoon sea salt

Directions

Step 1

Preheat oven to 350 degrees F (175 degrees C). Spray muffin cups with cooking spray.

Step 2

Heat olive oil in a skillet over medium heat; cook and stir spinach until wilted. Remove from heat and cool spinach. Squeeze spinach to remove excess moisture.

Step 3

Whisk egg whites and egg yolks together in a large bowl; add Parmesan cheese, Mexican cheese blend, garlic powder, sea salt, and spinach and mix well.

Pour egg mixture into the muffin cups almost to the top. Place the muffin tin on a rimmed baking sheet and pour water halfway up the sides of the muffin tin to create a water bath.

Step 4

Bake in the preheated oven until muffins are set in the middle, 20 to 25 minutes.

Nutrition Facts

Per Serving: 108 calories; protein 9.4g; carbohydrates 1.5g; fat 7.2g; cholesterol 71.6mg; sodium 228.4mg.

Low-Carb Chicken and Mushroom Soup

Delicious restaurant quality soup for those on the ketogenic/low carb diet.

Ingredients

½ cup butter

1 cooked chicken breast, cubed

1 small white onion, finely chopped

3 cloves garlic, finely chopped

1½ pounds fresh mushrooms, sliced

3 cups chicken stock

3 tablespoons chopped fresh tarragon, divided

salt and freshly ground black pepper to taste

2 cups heavy whipping cream

Directions

Step 1

Melt butter in a Dutch oven over medium-high heat. Add chicken; saute until lightly browned, about 3 minutes. Add onion and garlic; saute until softened, about 5 minutes. Stir in mushrooms; saute until tender, 5 to 10 minutes. Pour in chicken stock and 2 tablespoons tarragon; reduce heat to low. Season with salt. Cover and simmer soup until flavors are combined, about 25 minutes.

Step 2

Stir cream into the soup; cook until heated through but not boiling. Serve soup with pepper and the remaining tarragon on top.

Nutrition Facts

Per Serving: 531 calories; protein 15.3g; carbohydrates 8.2g; fat 50.2g; cholesterol 179.2mg; sodium 539.8mg.

Whole Wheat Oatmeal Strawberry Blueberry Muffins

I developed this recipe to add more fiber and develop a better diet.

Ingredients

1 cup whole wheat flour

1 cup oats

½ cup white sugar

2 teaspoons baking powder

½ teaspoon baking soda

½ teaspoon salt

1 cup milk

¼ cup vegetable oil

1 egg

1 teaspoon vanilla extract

2 cups diced strawberries

1 cup fresh blueberries

Directions

Step 1

Preheat oven to 425 degrees F (220 degrees C). Grease muffin cups or line with paper muffin liners.

Step 2

Mix flour, oats, sugar, baking powder, baking soda, and salt together in a bowl. Combine milk, vegetable oil, egg, and vanilla extract in a separate bowl.

Step 3

Stir milk mixture into flour mixture until batter is combined. Fold in strawberries and blueberries. Spoon batter into prepared muffin pan until full.

Step 4

Bake in preheated oven until a toothpick inserted into the center comes out clean, 18 to 22 minutes.

Nutrition Facts

Per Serving: 164 calories; protein 3.7g; carbohydrates 25.1g; fat 6.1g; cholesterol 15.3mg; sodium 245.4mg.

Vegan Sweet Potato Bread

Southern favorite that I modified for a vegan diet. This also freezes well.

Ingredients

1 cup chopped sweet potato

1½ cups white sugar

½ cup vegetable oil

1 over-ripe banana

1¾ cups sifted all-purpose flour

1 teaspoon baking soda

½ teaspoon ground cinnamon

½ teaspoon ground nutmeg

¼ teaspoon salt

teaspoon baking powder

1 cup water

½ cup chopped pecans

Directions

Step 1

Bring water to a boil in a large pot. Add sweet potatoes and cook until tender, 20 to 30 minutes; drain. Place sweet potatoes in a bowl and mash with a potato masher until smooth.

Step 2

Preheat oven to 350 degrees F (175 degrees C). Grease a 9x5-inch loaf pan.

Step 3

Stir sugar and oil together in a bowl until well mixed; beat in banana. Combine flour, baking soda, cinnamon, nutmeg, salt, and baking powder in a bowl. Alternate stirring the flour mixture and 1/3 cup water into the sugar mixture until combined. Mix in sweet potatoes and pecans; stir until batter is smooth. Pour batter into the prepared loaf pan.

Step 4

Bake in the preheated oven until top is golden brown, about 1 hour.

Cook's Notes:

Yams can be substituted for sweet potatoes, if desired.

The 9x5-inch loaf pan can be substituted with 2 small loaf pans.

Nutrition Facts

Per Serving: 295 calories; protein 2.6g; carbohydrates 44.2g; fat 12.7g; sodium 165.2mg.

Oven-Baked Beef Tagliata

This beef tagliata cooks in the oven and is perfect for those following a low-carb diet!

Ingredients

3 large cloves garlic, minced

2 teaspoons finely chopped fresh rosemary

1 teaspoon chopped fresh oregano

1 tablespoon sea salt, divided

2 teaspoons ground black pepper, divided

2 (1 1/2) pounds sirloin steaks, about 1 1/2-inches thick

1 tablespoon extra-virgin olive oil

6 cups loosely packed arugula

2 teaspoons extra virgin olive oil

1 teaspoon lemon juice

¼ lemon, sliced

2 ounces Parmesan cheese, shaved

Directions

Step 1

Place a cast-iron skillet in the oven and preheat the oven to 350 degrees F (175 degrees C).

Step 2

Combine garlic, rosemary, oregano, 1 1/2 teaspoons salt, and 1/2 teaspoon pepper in a small bowl. Rub spice mixture all over the steaks.

Step 3

Remove the skillet from the oven and add 1 tablespoon oil. Add steak and return to the preheated oven. Cook until steaks is browned on both sides, turning after 10 minutes, about 20 minutes total.

Step 4

Transfer steak to a cutting board and let rest for 10 minutes; then slice.

Step 5

Spread arugula on a platter and top with steak slices. Drizzle with 2 teaspoons olive oil and lemon juice and top with Parmesan cheese.

Nutrition Facts

Per Serving: 333 calories; protein 45.5g; carbohydrates 3g; fat 14.5g; cholesterol 86.3mg; sodium 1116.9mg.

Crustless Mini Quiche Lorraine

My favorite comfort food on a low-carb diet is this quick and easy crustless quiche. I make them with and without spinach, and sometimes double the amount of bacon, as the mood strikes me. This is a crustless, low-carb version of quiche Lorraine that I developed when my family switched over to a LCHF diet. Not intended for low-fat diets!

Ingredients

Nonstick cooking spray

1 (6 ounce) bag fresh spinach, finely chopped

1 (14 ounce) package cooked bacon, chopped

3 tablespoons dried chives

6 ounces Swiss cheese, shredded

8 large eggs

1 cup heavy cream

4 teaspoons salt-free seasoning blend

1 teaspoon onion powder

½ teaspoon garlic powder

freshly ground black pepper to taste

Directions

Step 1

Preheat the oven to 350 degrees F (175 degrees C). Lightly spray a 12-cup standard muffin tin with nonstick spray.

Step 2

Spray a skillet with nonstick spray. Saute spinach over medium-low heat just until wilted, about 3 minutes. Remove from heat.

Step 3

Divide bacon among the muffin cups. Squeeze moisture out of the spinach and place on top of bacon. Sprinkle with chives, then top with equal portions of Swiss cheese.

Step 4

Blend eggs, cream, seasoning blend, onion powder, garlic powder, and pepper in a mixing bowl. Pour mixture slowly into each cup, stopping just before it reaches the top.

Step 5

Bake in the preheated oven until a knife inserted in the center comes out clean, about 25 minutes. Remove from the oven and let rest for 5 minutes before serving; it's normal for puffy quiche to settle and flatten.

Cook's Notes:

Leftovers can be refrigerated. Reheat in microwave, 30 seconds to 1 minute, depending on your microwave.

Please note that substitutions may change the taste, texture, and carb content of the dish, so be sure to make adjustments if you use half-and-half instead of heavy cream, etc. I've used turkey bacon with good results, but regular bacon is best for a LCHF diet.

Nutrition Facts

Per Serving: 353 calories; protein 21.1g; carbohydrates 2.8g; fat 28.5g; cholesterol 200.6mg; sodium 856.8mg.

Conclusion

Metabolism is the sum of all catabolic (break down) and anabolic (synthesis) reactions in the body. The metabolic rate measures the amount of energy used to maintain life. An organism must ingest a sufficient amount of food to maintain its metabolic rate if the organism is to stay alive for very long. Catabolic reactions break down larger molecules, such as carbohydrates, lipids, and proteins from ingested food, into their constituent smaller parts. They also include the breakdown of ATP, which releases the energy needed for metabolic processes in all cells throughout the body. Anabolic reactions, or biosynthetic reactions, synthesize larger molecules from smaller constituent parts, using ATP as the energy source for these reactions. Anabolic reactions build bone, muscle mass, and new proteins, fats, and nucleic acids. Oxidation-reduction reactions transfer electrons across molecules by oxidizing one molecule and reducing another, and collecting the released energy to convert Pi and ADP into ATP. Errors in metabolism alter the processing of carbohydrates, lipids, proteins, and nucleic acids, and can result in a number of disease states. Certain foods may help slightly increase your metabolic rate, or how many calories you burn. So, consuming them regularly may help you lose weight and keep it off in the long term. However, these foods will not negate a high calorie or poor quality diet. For effective, lasting weight loss and weight loss maintenance, seek a gradual reduction in calories and choose mostly whole, minimally processed foods.